Allen Carr

The easy way to

quit caffeine

T0221600

Allen Carr

The easy way to
quit
caffeine

Dedication

To Colleen Dwyer, an amazing, exceptional person and a "TOP GUN" Allen Carr's Easyway therapist

This edition published in 2019 by Arcturus Publishing Limited
26/27 Bickels Yard, 151–153 Bermondsey Street,
London SE1 3HA, UK

DA005508UK

Printed in the UK

CONTENTS

ABOUT EASYWAY

Allen Carr's hundred-cigarettes-a-day addiction was driving him to despair until, in 1983, after countless failed attempts to quit, he finally discovered what the world had been waiting for – the EASY WAY TO STOP SMOKING.

His network of centres now spans the globe, operating in more than 150 cities in over 45 countries. Contact details for these centres are given at the end of this book.

The centres offer a genuine money-back guarantee based on which the success rate is over 90 per cent. The Easyway method is also available in regular book form, e-book format, CD audio book, digital audio book, webcast seminar, video on demand, iPhone + android apps, and DVD.

For details of these items, and other books which successfully apply Allen Carr's EASYWAY method to 'alcohol', 'weight control', 'fear of flying','worry', 'debt', and 'gambling', visit www.allencarr.com

INTRODUCTION

For a third of a century, Allen Carr chain-smoked 60 to 100 cigarettes a day. He'd tried all the conventional methods of quitting, including willpower and nicotine replacement, plus a variety of other substitutes and gimmicks, but nothing worked.

As he described it: "It was like being between the devil and the deep blue sea. I desperately wanted to quit, but whenever I tried I was utterly miserable. No matter how long I survived without a cigarette, I never felt completely free. It was as if I had lost my best friend, my crutch, my character, my very personality.

"In those days I believed there were such types as addictive personalities or confirmed smokers, and because my family were all heavy smokers, I believed that there was something in our genes that meant we couldn't enjoy life or cope with stress without smoking."

Eventually he gave up even trying to quit, deciding it was a case of once a smoker, always a smoker. Then he discovered something which motivated him to try again:

"I went overnight from a hundred cigarettes a day to zero, without any bad temper or sense of loss, void or depression. On the contrary, I actually enjoyed the process. I knew I was already a non-smoker even before I had extinguished my final cigarette and I've never had the slightest urge to smoke since."

It didn't take Allen long to realize that he had discovered a method of quitting that could enable any smoker to quit:

* EASILY, IMMEDIATELY AND
  PERMANENTLY
* WITHOUT FEELING DEPRIVED

* WITHOUT USING WILLPOWER,
  SUBSTITUTES OR OTHER GIMMICKS
* WITHOUT SUFFERING DEPRESSION OR
  WITHDRAWAL SYMPTOMS
* WITHOUT GAINING WEIGHT

After trying out the method on smoking
friends and relatives with spectacular results,
he gave up his successful career in the
financial world to devote himself to helping
other smokers quit.

He called his method "EASYWAY", and so
successful has it been that there are now
Allen Carr's Easyway clinics in more than
150 cities in 50 countries worldwide. Best-
selling books based on his method are now
translated into over 40 languages, with more
being added each year.

It quickly became clear to Allen that his
method could be applied to any form of
addiction. It has helped tens of millions

of people quit smoking, alcohol, and other drugs, as well as to stop gambling, overeating and overspending.

The method works by removing the sense of deprivation that addicts suffer when they try to quit with other methods. It removes the feeling that you are making a sacrifice.

This book applies the same method to the issue of caffeine addiction and, unlike other methods, it does not require willpower.

Too good to be true? I assure you that all you have to do is read the book in its entirety, follow all the instructions, and you will become free.

I'm aware that many people, who are unfamiliar with the method or those who have stopped by using it, assume some of the claims made about it are far-fetched or exaggerated. That was certainly my reaction when I first heard them. I was incredibly fortunate to attend Allen Carr's stop-smoking clinic in London in 1997, yet I did so under duress. I had agreed to go, at the request of my wife on the understanding that when I walked out of the clinic and remained a smoker she would leave it at least twelve months before hassling me about stopping again. No one was more surprised than I, except perhaps my wife, that I left the clinic already free from my 80-cigarettes-a-day addiction.

I was so inspired that I hassled and harangued Allen Carr and Robin Hayley – then MD, now Chairman of Allen Carr's Easyway – to let me get involved in their quest to cure the world of smoking. I was incredibly fortunate to be able to convince them to allow me to do so.

Being trained by Allen Carr and Robin Hayley was one of the most rewarding experiences of my life. To be able to count Allen as not only my coach and mentor but also as my friend was an amazing honour and privilege.

Allen Carr and Robin Hayley trained me well. I went on personally to treat more than 30,000 smokers at Allen's original London clinic, and became part of the team that has taken Allen's method from Berlin to Bogota, from New Zealand to New York, from Sydney to Santiago.

Entrusted by Allen with ensuring his legacy achieves its full potential, we've taken Allen Carr's Easyway from videos to DVDs, from clinics to apps, from computer games to audio books, to online programmes and beyond.

We've a lot of work to do, with so many addictions and issues to apply the method to, and this book plays a special part in our mission.

The honour of updating and developing Allen's method for this book has fallen to me and the amazing Colleen Dwyer, one of the most senior Allen Carr's Easyway therapists in the world. Colleen has played a vital role in the global success of Allen Carr's Easyway, and her talent and expertise have played a key part in the development of this book.

Developing Allen's work in this way means the most up-to-date, cutting-edge version of his method has now been applied to a whole host of issues.

Follow Allen Carr's instructions and you'll not only find it easy to become free from caffeine, but you'll actually enjoy the process. You won't just be free; you'll be happy to be free. That might sound too good to be true, but read on. You've got absolutely nothing to lose and everything to gain.

John Dicey, Global CEO & Senior Therapist,
Allen Carr's Easyway

THE EASY WAY TO QUIT CAFFEINE

Most caffeine drinkers are convinced that it's difficult to quit. The problem, we're told, is not only the physical withdrawal but also that we need to use willpower to resist the craving.

The wonderful news is that there is an easy way by which any caffeine addict can quit easily, immediately and permanently. You will not have to use willpower, suffer withdrawal pangs or need substitutes. I know you might find this difficult to accept, but it's true.

I've been proving it for over 30 years with my books covering a whole range of addictions and issues. They've sold a total of more than 16 million copies so far almost entirely on the basis of personal recommendation – with people who have escaped from their addiction happily passing news of the method on to others.

This book will provide you with an inspiring companion and enable you to stop consuming caffeine – easily, painlessly and permanently.

Let this be the first day of an exciting adventure, the day you start preparing yourself to be free. All you need to do is follow the instructions.

In fact, your first instruction is:
FOLLOW ALL THE INSTRUCTIONS

You could spend a lifetime trying to break into a safe and still not succeed. But if you know the correct combination or have a key, it's ridiculously easy. Lose the key or miss one part of the combination and you'll remain trapped.

THE KEY TO SET YOU FREE

This book contains the key, the combination of information you need in order to become free. It will enable you to escape.

Your second instruction is:
DO NOT QUIT OR CUT DOWN UNTIL YOU HAVE FINISHED THE BOOK

Please do not try to cut down or stop consuming caffeine until you have read the whole of this book. Just carry on consuming caffeine, whenever you want, as much as you want, until that point.

You might find that a strange instruction, but it's important.

To find it easy to quit, you must achieve a frame of mind whereby, whenever you think about any caffeinated product, you feel a sense of freedom and relief that you don't consume it anymore.

That's the only way to become, and remain, truly free.

Changing, or more accurately correcting, your perception of caffeine will actually be an exciting, eye-opening, and positive experience. No doubt you find that hard to believe, but read on – you have absolutely nothing to lose and everything to gain.

In the meantime, the third instruction is:
START OFF IN A HAPPY FRAME OF MIND

The fourth instruction is:
THINK POSITIVELY

Cast aside all feelings of doom or gloom. There is no need to be miserable. You are about to achieve something marvellous. See your journey through this book for what it really is – an exciting challenge.

Just think how proud you'll feel when you're free.

The fifth instruction is the most difficult to follow:

KEEP AN OPEN MIND

NEW THINKING

I can't over-emphasize the importance of keeping an open mind.

Some people believe my method is a form of brainwashing.

Nothing could be further from the truth. But it does involve counter-brainwashing and the reversal of beliefs that you may have held your entire life.

Question what you think you know about caffeine. Question what society and convention have led you to believe to be true. If you do that and follow the instructions, you cannot fail.

A QUESTION OF CHOICE?

Do you consume caffeine out of choice? It would seem so. You are the one who selects it in the store or café, pays for it, and puts it into your body. But are you really acting out of free will?

THE GREAT CAFFEINE CON

If a friend appeared to be getting good returns from an investment, you might be tempted to join them and invest yourself. If it turned out to be a confidence trick resulting in you and your friend losing all your money, would you regard that loss as being incurred through having made a genuine choice?

The fact is that you originally invested in the scheme based on phoney information. You continued to invest based on the same. You didn't choose to lose your money; you were conned.

Your consumption of caffeine is the result of a similar confidence trick. You made a decision to start consuming it based on flawed information.

You continued to consume it based on the same misinformation combined with addiction. You chose to have those first experimental cups of coffee or cans of drink, but after that you felt compelled to carry on. Your choice was taken away.

If you believe you genuinely choose to consume caffeine, why on earth would you need to read this book?

You could just choose not to consume it. But it's not quite as simple as that, is it?

WHO'S IN CHARGE?

You are reading a book about quitting caffeine.

If you wanted to quit playing golf, would you need to read a book on how to go about it?

The fact that you have experienced difficulties cutting back or ceasing to take caffeine indicates that you are not exercising control or choice.

MASS CAFFEINE CONSUMPTION

Over 80 per cent of adults in the UK use caffeine every day. At what point in your life did you consciously decide to consume caffeine every day and begin to feel uneasy if you didn't?

Every single day for the rest of your life is a pretty big commitment to something that you don't really need and something that costs you in terms of time, health and money.

In fact, you never chose to become – or to remain – a caffeine addict; no one chooses to poison themselves with a toxic liquid.

You just got sucked into it like every other caffeine addict on the planet.

Don't panic about being an addict. The addiction is actually easy to break once you know how.

HOW DO YOU TAKE YOUR CAFFEINE?

How do you consume caffeine? Most likely it will be from one or more of these sources: Precise levels of caffeine in each of these products are not easy to determine due to variations in the manufacturing process. This is just a general guide.

Coffee Serving	Expresso 30mL	Instant 237mL	Brewed 237mL
Caffeine in mg	47–75	27–173	95–200

Tea Serving	Black tea 237mL	Green tea 237mL	Ice tea 237mL
Caffeine in mg	14–70	24–45	11–47
Decaf	Tea	Coffee	Espresso
Caffeine in mg	0–12	2–12	0–15
Soft Drinks	Diet Coke 355mL	Mtn Dew 355mL	Normal 355mL
Caffeine in mg	23–47	42–55	23–35
Energy Drinks	Red Bull 248mL	5hr energy shot 60mL	Relentless 237mL
Caffeine in mg	75–80	200–207	75–80
Energy waters	approx. 75–80 per 237mL		
Energy gels	30–40mg in a 40g sachet		

"Health" drinks like Coke Life and Lucozade	26–39mg per 330mL
Chocolate contains wide variations but roughly	43mg in 100g
Medicines	130mg in a 2 tablet dose of headache medication
Diet products	50mg to 300mg per serving
Caffeine tablets	50mg of caffeine in each tablet

WHAT DO THE "EXPERTS" SAY?

Well, the latest advice from the European Food Safety Authority (EFSA) is that pregnant and lactating women, adolescents and people with liver problems should consume no more than 200mg a day.

But what about the rest of us?

MORE HARM THAN GOOD.

What are the experts actually measuring? Is caffeine harmful? Can the body take it?

My question is not about whether something can be tolerated by the body. My question is: "What is the point of taking it at all?"

For me, alarm bells start ringing when people justify something by minimizing the negatives.

I'm not asking, "Does caffeine do more harm than good?" I'm asking, "What good is there? What is the benefit?"

Guidelines like "consume no more than two cups a day" reinforce the idea of "a little bit of what you fancy does you good".

But there is no nutritional value in caffeine; by definition, it's pure junk. More importantly, it can easily be avoided.

TOLERANCE

With any addictive drug, you build up a tolerance to it, so let's say we take a view that 300mg a day is acceptable.

Will it stay at 300mg a day? Have you noticed your caffeine consumption creeping up?

Telling someone to limit their intake of an addictive drug is like telling someone that they can jump off the top of a cliff as long as they don't fall more than a few metres.

Your body can survive consuming junk, but that in itself is not a reason for doing so.

DO YOU WANT TO STOP?

Of course you do – that's why you're reading this book. I don't blame you. Caffeine does nothing for you. It's an addictive substance that benefits only the corporations selling it, and they're doing so in ever-increasing ranges of products.

Like any addiction, it keeps you coming back for more, so what's in it for you?

Maybe you've heard of studies claiming that caffeine provides all sorts of benefits, such as reducing the risk of Alzheimer's and improving memory and concentration.

Is that why you consume it?

CAFFEINE CRAZY

Did you have a fear of Alzheimer's (or memory and concentration loss) when you consumed your first "energy" drink or latte?

The fact is that caffeine doesn't reduce the risk of Alzheimer's. Nor does it aid memory or concentration. So what are your personal reasons for taking caffeine?

People give various arguments for it. We're curious, intelligent and like to think of ourselves as logical, so we want to make sense of things.

We therefore say things like:
"I like the taste and smell."
"It helps me concentrate."
"It gives me energy."
"It's sociable."
"It's a source of antioxidants."
"It helps me keep my weight down."
"It's a habit."

TASTE

Do you recall your first experience of the taste? It was probably a cup of coffee.

Most people remember that they really didn't like the taste. It's a bitter substance that tastes horrible. Your first experience of it was probably with milk and sugar to disguise the true taste.

Of course, these days youngsters suffer a double blow as their first experience of caffeine – most likely in the form of a so-called energy drink – is also laden with huge doses of sugar. It's a sweet sickly mess designed to mask the flavour of caffeine.

Sugar addiction? That's a whole different problem. If you still load your caffeine with sugar and milk or cream, then deep down inside you know your consumption has nothing to do with the taste. You're doing everything in your power to mask it.

The fact is that your brain has taught your body to cope with the foul taste, so you can get the drug to which you have become addicted.

SMELL

The smell of freshly brewed coffee can be lovely. But it's interesting that it's not alluring in the same way to non-coffee drinkers. It's just a lovely smell.

The only reason it triggers the desire for a cup of coffee is because we're addicted to caffeine. A rose may have a delightful smell, but that doesn't make us want to eat it. We love the smell of the ocean, but that doesn't make us want to drink it.

When has the smell of a lovely perfume ever made you want to consume it?

The fact is you don't consume caffeine because of the smell.

Once you've been freed from the addiction, you'll still be able to enjoy the aroma of coffee, but you won't feel compelled to drink it.

No more than you'd feel compelled to drink a cup of sea water during a walk along a sun-soaked beach.

Coffee really is the only caffeinated drink that smells strongly – tea doesn't and neither do so-called "energy drinks".

Your brain associates that smell with the next dose of your drug.

Once you're free from the addiction, the smell won't be a problem to you.

CONCENTRATION

You might think it helps you to concentrate, but in reality it does the complete opposite.

The fact is that as caffeine leaves your body it creates a very mild, empty, slightly insecure, slightly uptight feeling. It's incredibly mild – almost imperceptible.

But that feeling triggers the thought in your brain of: "I want a coffee" (or an "energy drink", or whatever form of caffeine you tend to consume). That thought creates a craving.

The mild, empty, insecure, slightly uptight feeling of caffeine withdrawal is now joined by a stronger, more noticeable craving for caffeine – a direct result of the thought – and a feeling of deprivation unless you satisfy that craving.

The more you crave it, the more distracting the feeling gets, and the more difficult you find it to concentrate on anything else. It's the ending of that aggravation you seek, when you have the coffee or caffeine drink that you mistake as being "an aid to concentration".

Imagine you were to undertake a challenging mental task – let's say a difficult crossword puzzle.

Now imagine how difficult it would be for you if a small child marched around the room kicking a tambourine and banging a drum. It would be almost impossible for you to concentrate.

There's no doubt that, were the boy to stop making a noise, you'd immediately be able to concentrate better than a moment before.

Yet would you conclude that the boy and his actions were an aid to concentration? Of course not.

Yet that is exactly the kind of credit you give caffeine when you claim it helps you to concentrate.

All you experience is the temporary ending of an aggravation caused by caffeine addiction. Caffeine causes the aggravation; it doesn't relieve it.

Caffeine withdrawal makes you feel restless and distracted.

That's not good for concentration.

ENERGY

This is THE BIG ONE for most caffeine addicts. The caffeine industry works hard and spends a fortune promoting the idea that caffeine gives us energy.

From birth we're surrounded by brainwashing suggesting the same.

We end up accepting it as fact without question.

The truth is that you were perfectly energetic before you started consuming caffeine.

Look at young children at a party running around like there's no tomorrow. That's a completely natural energy high and a completely natural emotional high.

Remember, this is before they're force-fed E-numbers and sugar-loaded jelly and ice cream. Before anyone had ever dreamed of any kind of so-called energy drink, young lads would play games of football lasting hours. They'd have a break for a visit to the water fountain before carrying on and playing on for hours more. Not a drop of caffeine in sight!

In fact, one of the saddest things about the modern-day caffeine trap, and for that matter the sugar trap, is that perfectly healthy, vivacious, athletic, and energetic kids are being conned into believing they have to drink caffeine-loaded "sugar bombs" to take part in sports or simple leisure pursuits.

As they get older, they're even conned into drinking the same kind of caffeine and sugar bombs with their first experiences of drinking alcohol.

The sight of school kids downing cans of "energy drink" on their way to school in place of breakfast is incredibly sad.

Even as an adult your natural state should be to feel energized anyway.

If you're not sick, you should have more than enough energy to enjoy whatever you want to do in life.

If you really are tired, then your body is asking for sleep and rest, not caffeine.

Taking caffeine is like taking out a payday loan. A quick injection of cash (energy) and they've got you hooked in, with interest, for the rest of your life, with you having to go back for more again and again and again until the day you do something about it.

The reality is that caffeine addiction makes you permanently tired and exhausted.

Take a look at anyone with a caffeine problem. They look tired, run-down, and ready to drop. The irony is that the only thing that's stopping them from returning to their energetic, athletic, vivacious former self is the one thing they think they need to function – caffeine.

For the few occasions in life when we need a little help to get through a late shift or to keep us going until the end of a long day, there are many natural, harmless, non-addictive and healthy stimulants to help temporarily carry us through.

The fact is, if you get caffeine out of your life you won't feel in need of any stimulants. You'll be brimming with energy.

IS CAFFEINE SOCIABLE?

It's you that's sociable, not caffeine! Caffeine doesn't chat, tell jokes or funny stories, listen to your problems, or make people feel comfortable.

In fact, the lie about coffee being sociable is laid bare merely by popping your head into any high street coffee bar. Most of the time, you'll see people queuing for coffee or sitting drinking coffee in silence, not saying a word to each other.

How sociable is that?

People talk about meeting at the coffee machine to justify their addiction to drinking coffee, but think about it.

We refer to "water cooler chat", meaning gossip that occurs when people bump into each other and engage socially by the water cooler in the office.

You can still bump into people by the water cooler (water is everything that coffee and caffeine products are not) and at the times when you genuinely want to get together with friends over a drink you have plenty of options that don't include caffeine.

And never forget – it's the situation that's sociable, not the drink.

THE NORM

The assertion that a reason for consuming caffeine is that it's the cultural norm would be amusing if it wasn't so silly.

At one time it was the cultural norm to perform rain dances and to burn people accused of witchcraft.

The history of mankind is peppered with behaviour that, at one time, was considered normal, but is now clearly seen as bizarre or abhorrent.

The consumption of caffeine will one day be consigned to the history books. Future generations will wonder why on earth we inflicted it upon ourselves.

ANTIOXIDANTS

People didn't even know what antioxidants were until 1954. Now people use them as an excuse for all kinds of indulgence.

If it's antioxidants you're after, then you're better off eating grapes, strawberries, blueberries, apples or any of the other natural, healthy, nutritious foods that contain them.

Foods in their natural state contain a balance of nutrients for your body. Nature should be our guide. We know instinctively that processing coffee beans or tea leaves, extracting an addictive ingredient and consuming it, is ludicrous.

Contriving lame excuses for doing so makes us feel stupid. Being addicted to anything damages our self-esteem – we know deep down we're lying to ourselves.

HABIT

We don't do anything purely out of habit. "Habit" just describes the "auto pilot" element of our behaviour.

Do you dress, brush your teeth or eat out of habit? No. However, as we have been performing these tasks every day throughout our lives we have developed a routine around them.

If for any reason we want to change that routine or habit, we can do so without any problem at all. I've been in the habit of brushing my teeth before my morning shower ever since I can remember. It's become completely automatic.

Yet if I wanted to switch to doing so after my shower, it would be easy. We don't get into the habit of drinking coffee and then get addicted to caffeine. It's the other way around.

HOOKED

We get addicted to caffeine and then get into the routine, or habit, of consuming it at regular intervals.

Once your brainwashed perception of the drug has been corrected and you're free from the addiction, your previous "habit" of grabbing a coffee on the way to work might make you think about the subject, but it won't make you want to do it, nor will it require you to use willpower or make you feel deprived.

Remember, in the past when you attempted to cut down, control, or stop consuming caffeine, you didn't start by changing your perception of the drug.

Instead, you felt as if you were missing out on something that gave you a genuine pleasure or crutch. No wonder you failed.

This time it's going to be different. We are going to remove all the brainwashing and the illusions which made you feel as if you were making a sacrifice.

This time you won't even be tempted to start again.

WAKE UP AND SMELL THE COFFEE

So why do you continue to take caffeine?
What is the motivation?

If it's not the antioxidants, or the energy, or
the enhanced concentration, or the smell,
or the taste, or the sociability, or the habit, or
because it's the cultural norm, then why do
millions of people do it?

Why do you do it?

You fell into one of the most subtle traps that
man and nature have ever combined to lay.

SPECIAL MOMENTS

Most people consider certain occasions when they consume caffeine as more special than others. When do you have your favourite caffeinated drink?

The first one in the morning? The one at mid-morning break? The one after a meal?

The first one in the morning isn't any different from the third or fourth one in the day.

How can identical drinks appear so different? The drink never changes. But our perception of it does.

Special moments when we consume caffeine invariably occur after a period of abstinence, i.e. when we've gone without for a while. The longer the period, the more special it seems to be when we are finally allowed our little fix.

The other factor involved in most special moments is exactly that! Some moments are special in themselves.

Hooking up in a café with a friend for a catch-up, relaxing after a meal, chilling out with colleagues during a break from work, or taking a break from shopping – these are all moments of genuine pleasure.

When we consume caffeine at those times, we mistakenly give the credit for the pleasure we experience to the drug.

One of my closest friends told me about how, when she used to go on holidays as a child to her uncle's farm, she found the farmyard smelled disgusting. She quickly got over it and nowadays she finds that very same smell quite lovely as it conjures up magical memories. It's clear that her holidays as a child weren't good because of the smell but in spite of it.

Your breaks aren't enjoyable because of the caffeine, but in spite of it.

The smell of caffeine may well bring to mind pleasant associations, but not because the caffeine itself contributed to the experience.

So how does the addiction work? It can be frightening to admit that you're addicted to a drug, even one as socially acceptable and prevalent as caffeine, but thankfully the addiction is easy to break once you understand it.

The Little Monster
Caffeine is a physically addictive drug which means that, after you consume it, it creates physical withdrawal.

This withdrawal takes the form of a mild, empty, slightly insecure, slightly uptight feeling. It's so mild, it's almost imperceptible.

When you take another dose of the drug, that mild, empty, insecure feeling temporarily disappears, leaving you feeling normal again. In fact, you take each dose of caffeine merely to try to return to the feeling you had all the time before you became addicted.

It's like a little monster inside your body that feeds on caffeine. If you don't feed it, it complains. Feed it and the feelings disappear for a while only to return as the latest dose withdraws from your body.

When you break free from caffeine addiction, you're going to starve that little monster to death.

Don't worry, the physical withdrawal is very slight and getting rid of the little monster is easy provided you're in the right frame of mind and follow some simple instructions which I will provide later.

The difficulty is not the physical withdrawal itself but the fact that it acts as a trigger for the real problem:

The Big Monster
From birth we're brainwashed into believing that we get some kind of benefit or crutch from caffeine; that it helps us concentrate, increases our energy levels and productivity, that it helps us socialize and be more competitive in sport. The effect of the little monster seems to confirm this.

When you consume caffeine, that empty, insecure, slightly uptight feeling disappears for a while and you do feel less empty, less insecure and less uptight than you did a moment before.

Withdrawal makes us feel physically lethargic while mentally restless. It is distracting and therefore impairs concentration.

Each dose of caffeine seems to relieve these symptoms and we are therefore fooled into believing that we get a genuine pleasure or crutch from it.

It is this belief that creates the feeling of deprivation when we try to quit. And it is this feeling of deprivation which creates the cravings associated with caffeine withdrawal.

Remember, the physical withdrawal (the little monster) is very mild. It's the thought process that it triggers, aided and abetted by the brainwashing (the big monster), that causes the unpleasant cravings.

This method removes the big monster.

All you have to do then is starve the little monster to death by stopping taking caffeine and you will be free.

BRAINWASHING

The conditioning that we have all been subjected to since birth creates the big monster. We're taught to have a distorted view of caffeine from a very young age.

It's not just seeing our parents consuming it, plus the coffee and energy drink adverts, that warp our perceptions. Virtually the whole of society has a brainwashed view of caffeine.

Caffeine is seen as an affordable and accessible pleasure – sophisticated, sociable and enjoyable. It's seen as something that can boost our endurance at work or in sports; something that can be beneficial when consumed in moderation but may cause some small problems if taken in larger doses. In other words, it's viewed as an innocuous addiction that presents no real problems to the average user.

But the reality is something entirely different.

Caffeine is a bitter, addictive drug which is a naturally occurring insecticide in certain plants. It attacks the central nervous system.

Large corporations understand only too well the addictive nature of the drug and, like sugar, they are adding it to as many of their products as they can, often justified by the ludicrous assertion that it's just flavouring.

Have you ever tasted pure caffeine? It's a bitter substance, which tastes terrible. One of the worst aspects of the brainwashing is that our own failed attempts to stop, as well as those of others, make us conclude that it's very difficult to escape and that, even if we do manage to quit, we'll feel deprived for the rest of our lives.

No wonder we find it so hard to stop!

THE SIDE-EFFECTS OF CAFFEINE

Headaches

Lethargy

Calories (from the products it is mixed with)

Dehydration

Liver and other organ damage

Jittery, wired feelings

Irritability

Decreased insulin sensitivity

Raised blood pressure

Heart palpitations

Expense

Stained teeth

Insomnia

Limited attention span

Coffee breath

Low self-esteem as a result of being controlled by a drug.

Caffeine is recognized as a highly addictive drug. It is a naturally occurring insecticide of the coffee bean – or more accurately, coffee seed.

BEWARE POISON

Pure caffeine is extremely toxic. Incidents of youngsters being taken seriously ill, and in some cases dying, from taking pure caffeine powder are sadly becoming more frequent.

Seemingly harmless caffeine products such as energy drinks are also causing serious problems. A 2014 study from the American Heart Association indicated that 40 per cent of the 5,156 calls to poison centres for "energy drink exposure" involved children under the age of six.

In most cases, the parents didn't know the children had drunk an energy drink. Many of the calls indicated that the children were suffering serious side-effects, such as abnormal heart rhythms and seizures.

BE CAREFUL

Pharmaceutical grade caffeine comes
with the following message: "WARNING!
MAY BE HARMFUL IF INHALED OR
SWALLOWED. INHALATION CAUSES
RAPID HEART RATE, EXCITEMENT,
DIZZINESS, PAIN, COLLAPSE,
HYPERTENSION, FEVER, SHORTNESS
OF BREATH. MAY CAUSE HEADACHE,
INSOMNIA, NAUSEA, VOMITING,
STOMACH PAIN, COLLAPSE AND
CONVULSIONS. FATALITIES HAVE BEEN
KNOWN TO OCCUR."

Of course, you're extremely unlikely to have
experienced the symptoms described in
these extreme cases.

However, it's important that you start to see
caffeine as it really is, rather than as society
generally regards it. After all, if it were
harmless, you wouldn't be reading this book.

CUTTING DOWN

Cutting down or trying to control an addiction doesn't work. It takes tremendous willpower and makes the drug appear more precious, just as dieting makes food appear more precious. You find yourself wishing your life away waiting for your next fix. In addition to that, you're causing yourself to suffer withdrawal pangs.

When you do finally indulge yourself, the relief – both physical and mental – is increased, so the illusion of pleasure is also increased and you become more psychologically addicted. Eventually your willpower runs out and you usually end up consuming even more caffeine than before.

In fact, the situation is far worse than it first appears. Because caffeine is a poison, the body develops a tolerance for it. In the early days when we're learning to consume it, all we're really doing is teaching our brains and bodies to cope with the foul taste of the poison. After a while, the body begins to tolerate it. Indeed, such is the brainwashing that we end up actually believing we enjoy the taste.

This process is double-edged. On the one hand, it means you can consume caffeine without it seeming unpleasant; but it also means that you don't completely relieve the withdrawal symptoms with each fix.

This is why, as we go through life, the natural tendency is to consume more and more. The more you imbibe, the more your tolerance develops, and the more you feel you need.

If you can recall your first shot of caffeine – whether it was a coffee, tea, energy drink or whatever – you will probably remember that it tasted foul.

You may also remember that it made you feel jittery and on edge. You certainly would not have imagined that, years later, you would feel so dependent on it that you would be reading a book on how to quit.

However, when that caffeine started to leave your body, you began to get that insecure feeling. It's so slight that you would not have even been aware of it. If you have another dose of caffeine within that withdrawal period, you get an immediate boost. The empty insecure feeling disappears and you feel better than you did just a moment before.

However, that subsequent dose of caffeine now leaves your body and again you experience that empty, insecure feeling of caffeine withdrawal.

The lifelong chain has started.

Once we're addicted, we receive a boost whenever we take a hit of caffeine. This is not just an illusion. We do actually feel better than a moment before. What we don't realize is that all we are doing is consuming caffeine to feel like a non-caffeine addict – to feel how we felt before we had our first-ever shot of the drug.

We are now constantly undergoing the empty, insecure feeling created by caffeine withdrawal.

Each time we experience that partial relief when we take caffeine, it reinforces the brainwashing and perpetuates the illusion that we get some kind of pleasure or benefit from it.

The worst thing that happens is that it begins to dawn on us that we no longer take caffeine when we choose to or want to, now we have to consume it every day. And the mere thought of not having it can create panic. Although we may try to block our minds to the fact, we instinctively sense that something evil has taken possession of us.

But no matter how much the drug drags you down, you still get that slight boost when you take it.

In John Steinbeck's *Of Mice and Men*, Lennie worshipped George because George saved him from drowning. It never occurred to Lennie that it was George who pushed him to jump into the dangerous river in the first place. It's the same with caffeine. In fact, the lower the drug drags us down, the more grateful we are for the little boosts it seems to give us and the more dependent we feel on it.

You cannot be truly happy as an addict. You can only be truly happy once you are free.

I promise you that, with the right approach, it takes no willpower. You can be happy and relaxed about quitting and enjoy the process. It takes no willpower at all to avoid watching a movie that doesn't interest you. That's what it's like when Easyway sets you free.

WHAT ABOUT KEEPING THE SPECIAL ONES?

The problem is not the caffeine itself; the problem is the brainwashing.

If you think that the occasional coffee, tea or energy drink provides some sort of pleasure or benefit, then you haven't seen through the illusion and you'll see a million doses in the same way.

MAYBE I'LL QUIT TOMORROW

So when will you stop consuming caffeine?

After you spend £20,000 ($26,500), the average amount a caffeine addict spends on caffeine in a lifetime?

Does that sound like an inflated figure? Research indicates that a heavy coffee drinker consumes more than 21 cups each working week, forking out as much as £2,000 ($2,650) a year on cappuccinos, lattes and espressos. And even the average consumer spends around £500 ($660) a year.

Hasn't caffeine already become an obvious problem for you? How many years have you been consuming caffeine? Do you ever ask yourself why you keep doing so?

It's time to stop putting off the day you quit. Why would you want to do that?

All we have to do is remove the brainwashing and understand the true nature of the trap.

Maybe you're resistant to the idea that you're an addict? Really! If that's the case, why on earth would you be needing to read this book?

HIGH OR LOW

Does caffeine give you a high or a low?

Everyone is falling over themselves to say caffeine gives you a high or a boost. Look at the words we use when we talk about it: *Energy* drink; Caffeine *Shot*; Red Bull gives you *wings*; Caffeine *jolt*; *Wired*; *Buzz*

Paradoxically, the impression that it provides a boost comes from the reality that caffeine creates a low. All the time that you are experiencing caffeine withdrawal, you are being kept in a low, fidgety, lethargic state. By taking more of the drug, you receive a brief boost as the new dose of caffeine temporarily curbs the withdrawal.

Each shot of the drug, far from ending the withdrawal, ensures that you'll undergo it again and again and again.

WHAT DO PEOPLE SAY WHEN THEY'RE DOING THEIR DRUG?

I need my caffeine hit.

We misunderstand the effects of caffeine on our system and then construct a whole belief system around our behaviour.

This is the brainwashing.

We buy into the idea of energy boosts, needing caffeine to stay awake or to concentrate, needing caffeine to socialize, wake up, or even to relax.

Caffeine starts to feel like a vital part of our existence.

When we're not consuming caffeine, we are withdrawing from it. In fact we're withdrawing from it even when we are consuming it because, as previously explained, it never completely relieves the slightly low physical state of emptiness and restlessness which it creates.

The brainwashing is exploited by the caffeine industry, which is more than happy to reinforce the illusions via advertising and marketing campaigns.

"IT GIVES YOU WINGS"

The emergence of premium energy drinks was largely led by Red Bull. Remember the first time you saw it for sale in a store.

"What an odd-sized can!"

"It costs how much? Really! It isn't even alcoholic! There must be something to it. I'll try it."

"Ugh – disgusting! There MUST be something special about it or people wouldn't buy it!"

These days Red Bull has crept its way into our pubs and clubs as a popular mixer with hard liquor. A veritable bomb of alcohol, sugar, and caffeine!

Whether it's vodka and Red Bull or the widespread "Jäger Bomb" (a shot glass of Jägermeister dropped into a glass of Red

Bull), there seems to be no stopping the march of caffeine products.

The product names are revealing: Monster, Relentless, Red Bull and Rockstar to name just a few. All aggressive, macho, sexy-sounding brands targeting impressionable youngsters.

Mixing energy drinks with alcohol seems particularly absurd. On the one hand, the energy drink is packed with caffeine and sugar (both stimulants), and on the other hand alcohol is a depressant. So we're simultaneously taking drugs whose effects counteract each other.

The marketing of energy drinks that have flooded into pubs and bars is equalled by that of those which have crept on to our sports fields. In spite of a complete lack of evidence that energy drinks provide any kind of performance enhancement, a generation of youngsters has grown up to believe that the only bottle worth having in your hand during a time-out is one containing a so-called "sports drink".

It's been interesting to see professional athletes, presumably after a bit of scientific research, moving back to drinking water to rehydrate and eating bananas to get an energy boost during games.

Yet the industry is unstoppable. Red Bull for example sponsors cool and fun events. Extreme sport seems to be its thing and its website looks more like a travel or sports website than one that promotes a synthetic, caffeinated, drug drink.

Red Bull doesn't just sponsor a Formula One racing team, it owns one. It bought a Major League Soccer team and renamed it the New York Red Bulls. It has pioneered a new model of advertising and marketing by conceiving, financing and producing extreme stunts like Felix Baumgartner's 24-mile freefall to Earth from space.

Its investment in sports is designed to promote an image of energy, daredevilry and heroism which becomes associated with its products.

This is a worrying strategy designed to appeal to youngsters at an impressionable age and get them hooked for life.

They're laughing all the way to the bank.

And putting ideas in our heads

"LOVING CUP"

I always thought of coffee as a sophisticated drink and tea as a working-class drink. Why? Were my perceptions being played with?

Was the caffeine industry working to capture every type of person and situation somehow?

I associated cool Italian chic with espressos and tea with a bunch of PG Tips monkeys! No one talks about "builder's coffee".

Can you remember the Nescafe or Kenco coffee advertising campaigns? The epic love affairs played out in ad-break episodes?

COFFEE CULTURE

What is society's perception of caffeine?

"One of life's little pleasures"
"Nothing to worry about"
"Sophisticated"
"Flavoursome mature person's beverage"
"Sociable"
"A stimulant that'll perk you up"
"Associated with the good life"
"Associated with a general need in the morning"
"Sexy, glamorous, cool, sporty, energy-giving, etc."

It's become all things to all people.

ENERGY

If you want a burst of energy, there are lots of things you can do:

Listening to your favourite song can be incredibly energizing

Exercising gets your heart pumping and blood flowing

Engaging your brain in a mental task, e.g. a crossword, creates mental energy

A brisk walk in the fresh air.

The fact is you don't actually need anything to take the place of caffeine. You haven't been getting any benefit from it anyway.

After the first few top-ups of caffeine, you remain just as tired, just as lethargic and run-down as you were in the first place.

If you look at people who seem to rely on caffeine to keep them going, you'll see this is true. They don't walk around with purpose; they're not bursting with energy. They normally look tired, run-down, lethargic and exhausted – as if they're running on empty.

Feeling tired or lethargic at times is perfectly natural, especially if you've had a late night or are working long hours. Listen to your body. Make sure that you get enough rest and enough good-quality sleep. The health benefits of doing so are immense and far-reaching, as are the negative effects of not doing so.

Of course there are occasions when we are required to push ourselves to work or play longer and harder without the opportunity for proper rest.

If you do feel tired or lethargic, a brisk walk in the fresh air can work wonders.

And remember, there are plenty of factors that could be causing you to feel tired at times. Starchy, carb-laden lunches can create problems with blood sugar levels during the afternoon, leading to lethargy and tiredness.

Once you're free from the toxin caffeine, you'll be far more inclined to take care about what else you put into your body.

If you feel tired, run down and lethargic, it's a sign that something is wrong. Look at how much sleep and exercise you're getting and try to eat foods that give you energy and keep you healthy.

CONFLICT

Mistakenly believing that caffeine gives you a genuine boost, rather than understanding that it makes you feel low, tired and drained, creates a mental conflict.

You end up convinced that the only way to energize yourself is to take caffeine. But at the back of your mind, you may worry about the health implications, the feeling of being controlled and the cost. You may therefore try to cut down on your intake.

This mental conflict is a hallmark of addiction. It creates a tug of war of fear that far outweighs the mild, physical withdrawal. On the one hand, fears that you can't cope with or enjoy life without your little pleasure or crutch; that you'll have to go through some terrible trauma to quit; and that, even if you do succeed, you'll have to spend the rest of your life feeling deprived and resisting temptation.

On the other hand, fears that it's poisoning you, costing you a fortune and controlling you. What the addict fails to grasp is that both these sets of fears are caused by caffeine.

Non-caffeine addicts suffer neither set of fears. You didn't suffer them before you got hooked and you won't suffer them once you're free.

POWER OF BRAINWASHING

All our lives we're subjected to brainwashing on all kinds of subjects. Our character and personality evolve as a result of nature and nurture, and there's often a blurred line between the two.

How can we have been raised to think that putting a paper tube of foul-tasting, addictive, burning leaves in our mouth and inhaling the smoke is a normal thing to do? From birth, we have been surrounded by people smoking, and so it has become normalized in our minds. The fact that smokers panic without cigarettes – and will go to virtually any length to obtain them if they run out – serves to confirm the illusion that they can't survive without them.

It's the same with caffeine. Roasting and grinding up a foul-tasting, addictive bean and then drinking it in a liquid solution is an extremely odd thing to do.

Those deepest in the caffeine trap openly admit that they feel they couldn't survive without their regular fixes. They often blame stressful, highly demanding jobs and long hours to justify their apparent dependence.

But which creatures would you say are most dependent on powerful bursts of energy?

What about the big cat family? Powerful super-hunters such as lions, tigers, cheetahs and leopards rely on surges of energy to catch their prey. And they do so without the need for caffeine.

Whether it's powerful hunters or animals that achieve feats of incredible stamina, we only have to look at the animal kingdom to see that we do not need drugs to survive, flourish and excel.

Before youngsters fall victim to sugar and caffeine addiction, we see them rushing around, playing games, racing each other and exploring without the need for any kind of so-called energy fix.

Look at the people around you. Although caffeine addiction is still rife, there are millions of ex-caffeine addicts and millions of people who've never been hooked in the first place. You'll find that they tend to be more energetic and stronger both physically and mentally than the addicts we know.

It sometimes makes us resent them because they prove to us that we don't need caffeine either, which makes us feel weak and stupid for not having quit ourselves.

You may still be finding what I'm saying difficult to take on board. Keep an open mind. Remember that everything I'm saying about caffeine is very good news because caffeine is very bad news indeed.

Scientists are discovering that it is far, far worse for us than we previously thought. In fact, it is hard to think of a single part of you that is not seriously and adversely affected by caffeine: it poisons every single part of your body, it creates depression and mood swings, and of course, as with all drug addiction, the slavery to it crushes your spirit.

A comprehensive list of the ways in which caffeine harms you would fill a small library. It is certainly beyond the scope of this little book. It is also beyond its remit. You already know that caffeine is making you suffer.

That's why you bought the book. Caffeine is doing plenty TO you. What may well be news to you is that it is doing nothing FOR you.

It doesn't help you relax or concentrate, it doesn't inspire you, it doesn't even give you real energy. What it does do, is put you in the state of body and mind that you would be in if a man-eating tiger suddenly appeared in the room.

That state would be very useful if a man-eating tiger did happen to be in the room; it is decidedly counter-productive when you are trying to clean the house, write an essay, negotiate a deal or complete your tax return.

And let us not forget that if there were a tiger in the room, your brain would naturally secrete exactly the right amount of the correct chemicals for you to deal with the situation in as efficient a way as possible.

These days most of us enjoy lives in which such dangers are few and far between. One of the modern equivalents of the dangerous tiger is the cut-throat business takeover. Would caffeine help you to have the edge in such a situation? Only if you gave it to your adversary!

There would already be enough adrenalin flowing in such a situation, caffeine would overload the system, and make you nervous.

Far from helping you to think clearly on your feet, this would impair your ability to see the situation with clarity and thus respond skilfully.

There was a famous experiment in which spiders were given various drugs. The object was to observe the varying types of web these spiders would weave on their respective drugs.

Interestingly, the craziest, most disorganized web of all was not, as you might expect, that of the spider on LSD or cannabis, but that of the spider on caffeine.

Perhaps you're thinking, "But I have written some excellent essays/negotiated great deals/cleaned the house from top to bottom/done some excellent presentations on caffeine." I don't doubt you have.

The key is in the story about the old man who snaps his fingers all day long on a street corner in New York.

A kid goes up to him and says, "Old man, why do you snap your fingers all day like that?"

The old man replies, "It keeps the tigers away."

The kid says, "But old man, there are no tigers in New York City!"

The old man snaps his fingers again and says, "See! It works!"

Of course you have been able to do these things well on caffeine. But is it because you were on caffeine, or despite that fact?

Let us not forget that caffeine, like nicotine, is an addictive drug. The main symptoms of caffeine withdrawal are headache, a fuzzy head, lethargy and difficulty concentrating.

Of course caffeine addicts feel more energized and able to concentrate once they've taken the drug. But this is not because of the active effect of the drug, which is to put the mind and body into a state of panic.

Panic never helped anyone think clearly. It is merely because the drug has temporarily suppressed the withdrawal symptoms that it creates.

As well as being a drug, caffeine is a powerful poison. Regular consumption of any poison makes the consumer very tired and run down.

Therefore, on top of the fact that withdrawal from the drug makes you lethargic in the morning, your base level of energy and well-being is brought right down by the systematic poisoning.

In fact, it is a triple low that you experience, and mistake for normal, in the morning.

Your "normal" is in fact the low of withdrawal, compounded by the low of your mental craving for the drug, compounded in turn by the depleted state of mind, body and spirit that every addict suffers and mistakes for normal.

These days the vast majority of us jump-start our systems with a Starbucks or a cup of instant before the day's work. The student gets his fix before he attends lectures or sits down to start his essay. He may take energy pills to stay up half the night and cram before his exams when he should be getting nourishing sleep, and on the potentially stressful day of the exam itself, he forces down this panic-inducing drug.

It is very common to see people being interviewed for jobs in Starbucks these days, just as it is common to see important deals being brokered there. The illusion is that caffeine oils the wheels, that the world turns on this drug, that human progress itself surfs on a vast sea of skinny "soyaccino"!

The reality is that we are a nation of burnt-out, exhausted caffeine junkies who have forgotten what it is like to enjoy genuine energy, and mistake a radical shock to the system for the real thing.

Bear in mind that consumption of caffeine has only been widespread for the last four hundred years or so.

Think about that. Chaucer wrote *The Canterbury Tales* without recourse to this drug. Michelangelo painted the Sistine Chapel as a result of his determination, hard work, skill, talent and drive without needing a single (let alone a double) "espresso"! Leonardo da Vinci didn't need a "Caramel Macchiato" to paint the *Mona Lisa* or *The Last Supper*, and the Roman Empire was built without a single "black Americano", "flat white", or can of "Monster".

And let's not forget that while it is true that there are no tigers in New York and it is true that the old man clicks his fingers, to link these two facts with the word "because" is an outright lie.

Let's keep in mind that the dizzy heights to which we have soared since we all started drinking coffee – such as the discovery of DNA, for example – were not reached because we were all drinking it, but despite the fact.

After all, if you take someone who has little or no aptitude in a particular area – let's say playing the guitar – do they suddenly

become a genius guitarist because they pour
a cup of coffee down their throat?

Isn't it obvious that if a person achieves
something extraordinary, it is because of
their genius, and despite the products they
consume, rather than the other way around?

The vast majority of human achievement
in the arts and sciences has been fuelled
not by caffeine but by genuine energy and
inspiration. These are your birthright. They
are inside all of us, and far from bringing
them out, caffeine will dampen them.

Unless you quit, of course!

The caffeine trap is a bit like someone who
hasn't got a broken leg buying a crutch that
is riddled with woodworm.

SO WHY DO WE DO IT?

Why do we continue to consume caffeine?
Caffeinated drinks don't even quench our
thirst.

We're almost force-fed caffeine as food
manufacturers mercilessly add it to the
most surprising foods: breakfast cereals, soft
drinks, chocolate bars, snacks, desserts – the
list goes on and on.

We're brainwashed into believing that it's
something we need as part of our everyday
life; that any time we feel down or tired,
there's a magic potion that will make us
feel better. The big monster is lurking in
our minds.

When we have caffeine for the first time, the
little monster is created.

Remember how the addiction works: the
first shot creates an empty, insecure feeling

and subsequent shots seem to take that feeling away. This is what awakens the big monster. We do feel better the moment we have another shot of caffeine, but it's just the ending of the dissatisfied feeling created by the drug itself. The longer the period of abstinence, the greater the sense of relief when we finally have our fix.

WHAT ABOUT THE PLEASURE?

Most of us experience caffeine for the first time in a way that makes tasting it almost impossible. It usually takes the form of tea or coffee whose taste is masked by milk and sugar. Even cocoa and hot chocolate, which contain relatively low levels of caffeine, are normally sweetened with sugar.

Give a child unsweetened tea, coffee or hot chocolate and they'll wince at the taste. It's only when we add milk and sugar that we can begin to find it remotely palatable. In fact, we never enjoy the taste which is why most people tend to obliterate it with additives. Eventually, we build up a tolerance to the foul taste, so we can get the drug into our body with the least aggravation. We either learn to cope without the milk and sugar because we know they're also bad for us and tend to make us put on weight, or we persist with sweetened, frothy cappuccinos or lattes which disguise the taste.

These days, energy drinks do much the same thing and they're trapping youngsters at an even earlier age. It pains me to see children on the way to school sipping oversized cans of energy drink as if it were the greatest thing on earth. By morning break they're often drinking more, then again at lunch break, and again on the way home.

Not only are these children subjected to caffeine addiction, they are often also suffering from malnutrition with a diet devoid of real, nutritious food, often high in sugar, salt, processed carbohydrates and fizzy drinks with little or no nutritional value.

Have you noticed that the profit-chasing food and drink corporations are increasingly adding addictive substances to their products? Maybe this is the first time you've thought about food and drink ingredients in these terms – as addictive additives.

As the food and drink giants bombard us with sugar, salt, caffeine and processed carbs, they not only make us increasingly obese but also ensure that we keep coming back for more by hooking us on their junk.

CAFFEINE WITHDRAWAL

Caffeine withdrawal symptoms are usually mild – an empty, slightly uptight, insecure feeling. There can also be fatigue and sometimes headaches. However, the physical withdrawal is not a problem. In fact, if you're in the right frame of mind, you can actually enjoy the purging process.

Drink a lot of water and, if necessary, take a headache pill that doesn't contain caffeine and you'll mitigate any discomfort.

THE COMEDOWN

Some people report feelings of mild depression and it's important to realize that this only occurs if you feel you're missing out on something, if you cling to the illusion that you're being deprived of a genuine pleasure or crutch.

If you're happy to be free and realize that there's nothing to give up so that you're not making any sacrifice whatsoever, then you can actually enjoy the process of escaping.

THE COST OF COFFEE

Maybe the cost is one of your motivations for wanting to quit caffeine? If you buy your coffee in high street coffee shops, it can add up to a significant amount each week, as can the amount spent on energy drinks.

Although it's great to save money as a result of escaping from the caffeine trap, try not to use that as a motivating factor. Instead view the money you save as a bonus. Quit caffeine for the simple reason that you'll enjoy your life more once free of your addiction.

That said, consider how much you spend on caffeine products per week. Now multiply that by 52. Now multiply that figure by the number of years you hope to live.

It's so easy to write off a few pounds a day. Being thousands of pounds a year better off is wonderful. The money you'll save over the rest of your life is a marvellous bonus.

ADDICTION CAUSES STRESS; IT DOESN'T RELIEVE IT

It never really dawns on us how hard we have to work because of our addiction.

We allow extra time on our journey to work in order to stop off to pick up our fix. We often have to queue. Sometimes we manage to be patient; at other times we get flustered and frustrated at people placing orders for breakfast sandwiches or pastries. This always seems to take an inordinate amount of time. While you wait. And wait. And wait.

Then the barista either doesn't remember your normal order (which annoys you seeing as you've ordered the same thing every day for years) or does remember your normal order (which – if you consider it for a moment – makes you feel a little uneasy).

Then they either ask your name (which annoys you again for the same reason it annoyed you when they couldn't remember your order) or write your name on the cup without asking (which again occasionally causes those pangs of concern).

They take your hard-earned money and then you queue some more. And wait. And wait.

It's at times like this that your mind might wander off to thoughts of junkies at a methadone clinic queuing for their fix or to the patients in the movie *One Flew Over The Cuckoo's Nest* queuing for their medication. Looking at a coffee queue during the morning commute, it's impossible not to feel compassion for the poor victims of caffeine. The relief on their faces is obvious as they escape from the queue and scurry on their way, clutching their fix.

When you don't manage to get your fix – e.g. you're running late – you have to contend with the headaches and the distraction and frustration of wanting caffeine but not being able to have it, and reach the point where any source of caffeine will do, no matter how foul-tasting.

What kind of pastime is this? We're either feeling lousy because we've had too much, or lousy because we haven't had enough! We eventually reach the stage where we're fed up with the whole business. We just want to escape. Isn't that why you're reading this book now?

We know we're in the grip of something that's doing us harm, costing us money and controlling our lives, and we hope one day we'll wake up and magically not want caffeine anymore.

But you can escape from this addiction easily, permanently and happily. All you need to do is make a decision to do so and follow some simple instructions.

You have reached a fork in the road. You can decide to continue pointlessly consuming caffeine for the rest of your life, obtaining no benefits at all, suffering the cost, the inconvenience, the slavery, the tiredness, the lethargy, the nausea and the withdrawal... or you can choose freedom.

STOP OR CUT DOWN?

Your original objective when you picked up this book may well have been to try to control your intake, to cut down on the amount of caffeine you consume rather than to cut it out completely.

Some people consider cutting down prior to cutting it out completely to be sensible. The idea is to wean yourself off caffeine gradually, thereby reducing the physical withdrawal symptoms when you do stop completely.

The problem with cutting down gradually is that it makes caffeine seem more precious rather than less.

Within minutes of starting a diet, the thought of food starts driving us to distraction when in the normal course of a day we might hardly even think about it apart from at mealtimes.

Combined with that "forbidden fruit" effect, as mentioned earlier, the shots of caffeine we consider as "special" normally occur after a period of abstinence – i.e. when we've not had any for a while.

Cutting down tends to make every shot of caffeine appear "special", so it can perpetuate the illusion that you're making a sacrifice.

In any case, as long as you understand that you're not giving anything up, withdrawal from caffeine is barely noticeable. Feeling a bit tired, anxious and having a headache isn't that far from normal, everyday life for even the lightest caffeine addict.

It's nothing that keeping hydrated with water and, if necessary, an aspirin or another caffeine-free headache pill and a little rest won't sort out.

Anyway, if there's no benefit to taking caffeine frequently then there's no point in taking it occasionally either. Attempts to cut down usually fail and our intake usually returns to its previous level or even higher.

There's only one way to control your caffeine intake and that's to stop taking it completely.

ILLUSIONS

Take a look at the two tables below, one square, one rectangular. Which table is longer?

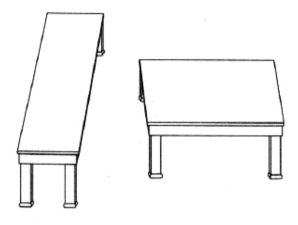

If I were to tell you that the dimensions of each table are exactly the same, you'd be extremely sceptical, wouldn't you? You've already accepted that it's one square table and one rectangular one because that's what I told you it is and it tallies with that you see.

However, the fact is they're both identical.

If you don't believe me, take a ruler and measure them. Extraordinary, isn't it? The reason I'm showing you this illusion is because I want to demonstrate how our minds can easily be tricked into accepting as true something that is false.

Your only frame of reference regarding caffeine is your addicted state of mind and body, so in that context, a shot of caffeine seems to deliver a boost. In reality, it's dragging you down mentally and physically.

The only reason you take caffeine is to try to get rid of the withdrawal – i.e. to feel like someone who doesn't take it, since they never experience withdrawal – and to feel like you felt the whole of your life before you got addicted to it. The only thing stopping you from feeling that way for the rest of your life is the next shot.

SO WHAT IF IT'S AN ILLUSION?

Illusions are normally fun. We love watching movies even though we know they're not reality. We all go through the masquerade of pretending we believe in Father Christmas because it's fun for the kids.

Most of us love to watch a magician even though we know we're not actually watching real magic. Illusions are great and it's healthy and fun to engage with them *when they make us happy.* But this illusion is not making you happy.

It's destroying your quality of life, making you feel ill and costing you a fortune.

THE INCREDIBLE MACHINE

We're given incredibly strong bodies. Unfortunately, we tend to treat them terribly. We smoke, take alcohol and other drugs, avoid exercise, overwork, deprive ourselves of sleep and gain weight. Some do all these and more for years. Some for decades!

Yet our bodies survive in spite of the abuse we subject them to. What an incredible piece of machinery the human body is!

And how very much stronger it is if treated with respect. Many addicts, who have consulted other types of therapists prior to coming along to our clinics, complain that they were questioned about their early childhood. They find this rather annoying because they can't see the significance of the questions. In one way, they are absolutely correct. In order to understand the addiction trap fully, you need to go back further – over three billion years, when life on this planet first developed. The human body is the result of three billion years of trial and error and is by far the most sophisticated and powerful survival machine on the planet.

When I was set free from my addiction to nicotine, it was as if I'd discovered an incredibly powerful machine: THE HUMAN BODY and in particular THE HUMAN BRAIN.

I firmly believe that this machine is better equipped to handle any situation without drugs.

When we're young, we're aware of the physical power and strength of that body, but as we grow a little older we become physically and mentally weaker. We know that our lifestyle is probably not helping. That we could eat more healthily, get more sleep and rest, avoid drinking too much or putting other toxins into our bodies.

But to an extent we've been brainwashed into accepting some kind of decline into old age, in some cases when we're not even out of our twenties!

Let's just pause a moment to consider the incredible sophistication of our bodies.

Can you do the ironing, make the bed, answer the phone, do the shopping and clean the car? Of course you can. But could you perform all these tasks at the same time?

Now consider the thousands of tasks that our bodies perform automatically, all at the same time, even as we sleep.

Our heart has to keep pumping, never missing a single beat. Blood must carry energy and nutrients to every part of our body.

Our internal thermostat has to maintain our body temperature at the correct level. Every one of our organs, including our liver, lungs and kidneys, has to continue to function in harmony with all the others. Our stomach must digest our food. Our intestines must distinguish between food and waste, extract the former and arrange disposal of the latter.

Any good doctor will tell you that your greatest ally in fighting infection and disease is not him or any drugs he can prescribe, but your immune system, which, while all the above functions are being carried out, automatically supplies chemicals such as adrenalin and dopamine to whatever part of your body needs them, at the right time and in the correct quantities. Our knowledge of the human body has expanded a thousand-fold in the last hundred years. We can transplant organs and achieve mind-boggling results with genetic engineering.

However, the greatest experts on these subjects admit that this increased insight into the functioning of the human body makes them realize how little we understand about the workings of that incredible machine.

All too often it has been shown that in the long run the interventions that we undertake with our limited knowledge cause many more problems than they solve.

If your highly sophisticated computer developed a fault, would you let a gorilla try to fix it? One scientist described unfolding knowledge about the workings of the human body so far as being like clearing a space of approximately 12-foot circumference in the centre of a huge forest. Clear just one more yard all round and you suddenly have a circumference of over 30 feet to clear. Clear just another yard and you are now confronted by a circumference of 50 feet.

The human body is by far the most powerful survival machine on the planet. It is a million times more sophisticated than the most powerful spacecraft made by mankind. If the oil in our car showed the slightest discolouration, we would have it changed. If we had treated our car as we have abused our bodies over the years, they'd break down and need to be scrapped immediately.

The human body is the culmination of over three billion years of trial and error, all designed to achieve one object and one object alone: SURVIVAL.

Three billion years is an awful lot of time for development and when so-called intelligent mankind contradicts the laws of nature, without knowing the exact consequences of his actions, HE IS CERTAINLY NOT BEING INTELLIGENT.

Our every instinct is to ensure that we survive. It's that instinct that has made you question your consumption of caffeine.

We think of tiredness and pain as evils. On the contrary, they're red warning lights. Tiredness is your body telling you that you need to rest. Pain is telling you that part of your body is being attacked and that remedial action is necessary.

We think of hunger and thirst as evils. On the contrary, they're alarm bells: your body warning you that, unless you eat and drink, you will not survive.

Each of our senses is designed to ensure that we survive. We're equipped with eyes to see danger, ears to hear danger, a nose to smell it, touch to feel hot or sharp surfaces and taste to know the difference between food and poison.

Many doctors now consider that drugs like Valium cause more problems than they solve. These drugs have a similar effect to alcohol. They take the person's mind off their problems, but they don't cure them. When the effect of the drug has worn off, another dose is required.

Because the drugs themselves are addictive poisons, they have physical and mental side-effects and the body builds an immunity to the drug so that its blocking effect is reduced.

The addict now has the original stress plus the additional physical and mental stress caused by feeling dependent on the drug that is supposed to be relieving the stress. Eventually, the body builds such an immunity to the drug that it ceases even to give the illusion of relieving stress. All too often the remedy is now either to administer larger and more frequent doses of the drug, or to subject the patient to an even more potent and dangerous drug. The whole process is an ever-accelerating plunge down a bottomless pit.

Some doctors still defend such drugs by maintaining that they prevent the patient from having a nervous breakdown in the short term. Again they focus on removing the symptoms. A nervous breakdown isn't a disease; on the contrary, it's a partial cure and another red warning light. It's nature's way of saying, "I can't cope with any more stress, responsibility or problems. I've had it up to here. I need a rest. I need a break!" The problem is that people often take on too much responsibility. Everything is fine while they're in control and can handle it. In fact, they often thrive on it.

However, everyone has phases in their life when a series of problems coincide. Observe politicians when they're campaigning to become president or prime minister. They are strong, rational, decisive and positive. They have simple solutions to all of our problems. But when they are elected, you hardly recognize them as the same person.

Now that they have the actual responsibility of office, they become negative and hesitant.

No matter how weak or strong we are, we all have bad patches in our lives. The usual tendency at such times is to seek solace through what we've been brainwashed into regarding as our traditional crutches: alcohol, nicotine and/or other drugs. It may be the usual thing to do, but there's absolutely nothing rational about it.

The only answer to stress is to remove the cause of the stress. It's pointless trying to pretend that the stress doesn't exist. Whether the stress is real or illusory, drugs will make the reality and the illusion worse.

Another problem is that we are also brainwashed into believing that we lead very stressful lives. The truth is that the human species has already successfully removed most of the causes of genuine stress.

We no longer have the fear of being attacked by wild animals every time we leave our homes and the vast majority of us don't have to worry about where our next meal will come from or whether we'll have a roof over our heads.

How would you like to be a rabbit? Every time you pop your head out of the ground you not only have the problem of searching for food for yourself and your family, but you have to avoid becoming the next meal of some predator. Even back in your burrow, you can't relax or feel secure as you're at risk from floods, ferrets and myriad other hazards.

The stress of serving in the Vietnam War understandably caused many servicemen to turn to drugs. But they served for a comparatively short period. How does a rabbit survive "Vietnam" its whole life, yet still manage to procreate at a prolific rate and feed its family? The reason that rabbits can take all this stress and trauma in their stride is because they have adrenalin and other drugs occurring naturally. They also benefit from possessing the powers of sight, smell, hearing, touch and instinct – in fact they have everything they need to survive. Rabbits are extraordinary survival machines, BUT HUMAN BEINGS ARE EVEN MORE EXTRAORDINARY.

We have reached a stage of evolution whereby we can partly control the elements themselves. Properly organized, we could virtually eliminate the effects of droughts, floods or earthquakes. We really have just one substantial enemy to conquer: OUR OWN STUPIDITY.

At our stop smoking clinics we ask smokers, "Do you have a smoker's cough?" Often the reply is: "I would stop smoking if I did." A cough isn't a disease. On the contrary, it's another of nature's survival techniques to eject harmful deposits from the lungs – just as vomiting is another survival technique to eject poisons from our stomachs.

Imagine being a pilot flying a plane over the Alps in blanket fog. You'd be entirely dependent on your instruments: altimeter, radar, speedometer, fuel gauge, compass, etc. Even if they were all functioning properly, it would still be a very scary business indeed, particularly if you had a fear of flying, as I once had.

You notice that your altitude has dropped to 8,000 feet. Knowing that the higher peaks are in excess of 16,000 feet, you wouldn't feel safe until you'd increased your altitude to above the tallest peak, plus a margin for error. What would you think of some idiot who said, "Why don't you just adjust the calibration on your altimeter to read 18,000 feet?" That would be even dumber than removing the oil-warning light rather than topping up the oil, or replacing a fuse with a nail because it kept blowing.

Taking a drug means that you are altering the calibration of one or more of your senses which are the instruments on which your well-being depends. A classic example is drinking and driving.

The biggest idiot on earth wouldn't dream of altering the settings on his altimeter if he was flying over the Alps in a blanket fog (or at any other time). Yet that is effectively what we do when we take drugs. The increased security, courage, confidence and happiness we experience when we free ourselves from addiction is truly priceless.

WHAT THE FUTURE HOLDS

With all addictions, it's not where you are *going to* that is important, it's what you are *escaping from* that counts.

"But nothing can beat sitting in your garden on a summer's morning with the sun shining and pouring a freshly made cup of aromatic coffee while reading the newspaper."

Well, there is something that beats that! Sitting in the morning summer sunshine enjoying your garden, reading the newspaper without the need or desire to consume an addictive, toxic substance that regularly makes you feel moody and suffer headaches if you can't have it, or makes you feel ill, tired, and generally lousy, and controls you, while costing you a fortune at the same time.

The real pleasure in that situation comes from the sunshine, and the warmth of it on your face. It comes from having a leisurely start to your day. It comes from enjoying the view of the garden, and reading the newspaper in absolute relaxation and peace.

The coffee has only ever been "sneaking a ride" on the back of these lovely components that make up the moment.

WHAT IS ADDICTION?

Don't get caught up with what other so-called "experts" say about addiction. They are unwittingly adding to the fear and confusion surrounding the subject.

Addiction is not an all-powerful mystical phenomenon or a permanent illness or condition that you can never free yourself from.

At its root is a simple misunderstanding. Your brain mistakes caffeine as providing relief from caffeine withdrawal rather than being the cause of it.

This back-to-front thinking allows the brainwashing to take root – i.e. the illusion that caffeine provides us with a genuine pleasure or crutch – and grow in our mind. This creates a feeling of deprivation when we try to cut down or quit.

YOUR FREEDOM FROM THE TRAP

To free yourself from this addiction requires a few basic corrections to your perceptions. Then you just have to follow some simple instructions.

THE FINAL SHOT AND THE INSTRUCTIONS

Do you feel ready to quit? By now you should be champing at the bit. If you're not, then please review the text again. It's perfectly natural to feel nervous, so don't be concerned if you are.

I have excellent news for you. You are about to consume the only caffeine that can bring you true enjoyment:

YOUR FINAL SHOT

Get it clear in your mind, there is nothing bad happening in your life today; there is in fact something wonderful happening. This is one of those rare occasions when you are making marvellous positive gains and losing absolutely nothing. There's a massive upside and no downside whatsoever.

So approach the process of stopping not with gloom or doom but with a feeling of excitement, of relief that your addiction is behind you, and of elation that you are finally free. Enjoy being free right from the moment you have your final shot.

Before you take your final shot of caffeine, I need to issue a warning. It's one thing to escape from the caffeine trap, but you need to ensure that you don't fall into it again. There are two main dangers and you need to be prepared for them both.

One is that you'll have a late night, or a run of late nights at work, or a heavy weekend that leaves you tired, run-down, and lethargic.

There will always be some helpful soul, with the best of intentions, that will try to force a coffee or caffeine drink down your throat. That shot of caffeine would re-trigger the addiction and restart the whole nightmare that you are now escaping from. It would ensure you feel tired, run down and lethargic for the rest of your life. Remember that.

The second danger is that because Easyway makes it easy to quit, you can fall into the trap of thinking, *"What possible harm can there be in having just one shot? Even if I did get hooked again, I'll find it easy to quit again."*

The moment you even start to ponder the thought of having just one shot, you are no longer following the Easyway method – so make a point of reminding yourself how lucky you are to be free and how miserable being a slave to caffeine made you.

Remember there is no such thing as just one shot. See it as it really is: the whole lifetime's chain.

Some people question the need for a final shot of caffeine. Perhaps it does sound contradictory for me to say that caffeine does absolutely nothing for you whatsoever, and then recommend you have a final shot.

I do so for good reasons. Not least of which is that the main difficulty in quitting is the doubt: when do you become free? It is important that you realize you will have achieved your goal the moment you finish your final shot – whether that be a can of energy drink, a double espresso, or a bucket-size cup of black Americano. The moment you finish it you are free.

Within a few days or weeks, you will experience either a sporting or social or stressful or tiring situation when previously you would have automatically turned to caffeine. Yet on this occasion it will suddenly occur to you that the need or desire to drink caffeine simply didn't even cross your mind. It's a wonderful moment when you know that you are free. I call it the MOMENT OF REVELATION. Don't wait for it to happen – just enjoy it when it does.

This is a very special day. We like to ritualize and celebrate special days like birthdays and weddings, and this is certainly one you will want to remember. So why not celebrate your last shot of caffeine?

Let's get it out of the way now so that you can be free for the rest of your life. Before you drink it, take time out to close your eyes and make a solemn vow, a commitment to yourself, that it will be your last-ever shot

of caffeine. Concentrate on the foul taste,
and ponder how you were once conned
into paying a fortune just to pour that filthy
poison down your throat.

GET ON WITH ENJOYING YOUR LIFE!

Having made what you know to be the correct decision, NEVER EVER question that decision. This is one of the key differences between Easyway and the willpower method. The difficulty in quitting lies not in the physical withdrawal pangs, but in continuing mentally to crave the drug and in questioning or doubting your decision never to take it again.

Some decisions in life are difficult. We have to weigh up the pros and the cons. But there are no pros whatsoever to consuming caffeine. If you begin to question your decision, you will start to crave caffeine. You will feel miserable and deprived if you don't have any and you will feel even more miserable if you do.

1. There are many people who have a huge vested interest in ensuring you never escape from the caffeine trap. They

want to keep you scared and confused. Remember you're making a marvellous decision and one that you know is correct even as you make it. Challenge any argument in favour of taking caffeine again. Question any so-called "evidence" that seeks to support the illusion that it provides any genuine pleasure or crutch. Understand where that "evidence" comes from and in whose interest it's presented.

2. Don't think, "I must never have caffeine again." That would create a feeling of deprivation. Instead, start with the feeling, "Isn't it great! My life is no longer affected by caffeine. I'M FREE!"

3. Do not – I repeat, do not – try to avoid thinking about caffeine. Let me illustrate the futility of attempting to do that. I would like you not to think about a huge, pink elephant. What have you started to think about? It's impossible to deliberately

not think about something. In fact, the more you try, the more you think about it. In any case, there's no need not to think about it. There's nothing bad happening. It's *what* you're thinking that's important. If you think, "I'd love a coffee", or "I need caffeine", or "When will I be free?", you'll make yourself miserable. But if you think "FANTASTIC! I'M FREE!", you'll enjoy thinking about caffeine, and the more you think about it, the happier you'll be.

4. Be aware that for the next few days there will be a little monster inside your body, wanting to be fed. The feeling might register as just a slight, empty, insecure feeling, or just the feeling of "I want some caffeine". You may feel a little tired or lethargic or have a headache. Either way, don't worry about it. Remember, that is what you've been suffering ever since you fell into the trap and it is so slight we don't even know it's there most

of the time. The great news is that you know that little monster is dying. You're starving it of caffeine. Think of it as such. Any headaches or tiredness are all part of the monster's demands for caffeine. It is he who is dependent on caffeine, not you. Once you realize that he has lost his power over you, the situation is immediately reversed. You now control him. You are going to starve him of caffeine and revel in his death throes.

5. Don't worry if you occasionally forget that you've quit. By that I don't mean you can have the occasional shot. I mean don't panic if the thought "I'll have some" enters your mind. Or, if when someone asks if you want a coffee, you say yes on autopilot. At those times relax, confirm you just forgot that you quit, and feel good about being free. Don't feel foolish telling the friend who's getting you a coffee to cancel your order. They'll

understand and find it impressive that you managed to forget that you quit. It's not a bad sign. It's no different to hiring a car and turning on the windscreen wipers instead of the indicators because the controls are on opposite sides on the car that you normally drive. Before long you get used to it and it doesn't cause you a problem anymore.

6. Don't panic if you accidentally have caffeine. Take care to check the ingredients of soft drinks, medications and foods before you buy them. On the rare occasion that you might discover that you accidentally imbibed caffeine, just brush it off. Consider it like the rumble strip on the hard shoulder of the motorway. A warning to take more care and keep clearly in mind the fact that you "got away with it" does not mean it's possible for you to have the occasional shot deliberately.

7. Don't wait to be a non-caffeine addict. You become one the moment you have your final shot. This is where people on the willpower method struggle. They think they have to take one day at a time or that somehow they have to survive for a certain amount of time before they can be free. You don't need to do that. Because you have got rid of the belief that caffeine provided you with any sort of benefit or crutch, you're free the moment you finish your final shot. Don't wait to be free – you already are.

8. Accept that like everyone else on the planet you'll have good days and bad days that are completely unrelated to having quit. You might feel tired after a late night out or a bit sluggish mid-afternoon after a run of tough days at work. Remember that's just your body reminding you to take enough rest or eat properly or avoid other addictive poisons. It's not a reason to take

caffeine. At such times, feel good about having escaped from the caffeine trap and focus on the fact that you'd feel ten times worse if you were still a caffeine addict.

9. Realize that you are in control of the craving and not the other way around. People often ask how long it takes for the little monster to die and for the cravings to end. The fact is that within a few days you'll feel a whole lot better. The headaches, the lethargy, the tiredness, and any feelings of insecurity or anxiety will have gone. Remember, those are the symptoms you suffered every day as a caffeine addict. Whether the thought, "I want a shot", is triggered by the little monster, or the fact that you momentarily forgot that you quit, or for any other reason, you are still in control. You have the choice of either reminding yourself that you are free from the whole nightmare, or starting to mope for caffeine. These are

wonderful moments to remind yourself how lucky you are to be free.

10. Don't mourn. If a friend or relative dies, you go through a period of mourning. No matter how great the trauma, time does begin to heal the wound and life goes on. But you are still left with a void that may never completely go.

When people quit caffeine by using willpower, they go through a similar mourning process. They know they'll be better off without it, but retain their brainwashed view of it. They believe they're giving up a genuine friend, pleasure or crutch and can remain vulnerable to the drug for the rest of their life. It only takes one bad day, late night, or tough week at work before they reach for their "old friend". In no time at all they end up back in the trap.

However, if your mortal enemy dies, there's no need to mourn. In fact, it's a cause for celebration and you can rejoice for the rest of your life. It's your choice. You can spend the next few days moping because you can no longer have caffeine; or for the rest of your life, whenever the subject of caffeine crosses your mind, you can think: FANTASTIC! I'M FREE!

11. Don't change your life in any other way purely because you quit caffeine. If you enjoy meeting friends in a café during breaks from work or shopping, then carry on doing so. When you use willpower to quit caffeine, those can be difficult moments when you feel deprived and envious of others. With Easyway, you will be able to relax, enjoy the company of your friends and feel great about being free.

12. Resist the temptation to convert your friends. Once you're free, it's only natural to want to help your friends escape too. But even good friends can become very defensive if they feel they are being preached to or judged. Far better to have them inspired by the ease with which you carry on life as normal without being bothered by caffeine. When they see you full of energy and perfectly able to cope with the stresses and strains (and late nights) of life without the need for caffeine, they'll be inspired to ask you how you got free. They'll be far more receptive at that point than if you attempted to convert them directly.

13. Don't use substitutes. Of course there will be times when you want a drink and previously at that time you might have felt compelled to have a caffeinated one. Of course at such times you should feel free to have a non-caffeinated drink.

But be wary of any thought process that implies any sense of deprivation. So rather than think, "I can't have a coffee, so I'll have a herbal tea instead", make sure that you remind yourself how lucky you are to be free. The thought "Great, I'll have a herbal tea" is empowering, reaffirming, and positive. Don't worry if initially the former thought occurs and if it does, just make sure you correct the thought to the latter.

After quitting caffeine with this method, the thought of drinking something that tastes like whatever your fix was, such as decaffeinated coffee, is unlikely to appeal.

Unlike previous attempts to quit or cut down, you won't feel deprived of caffeine so you won't feel the need to substitute. But clearly you'll get thirsty at times, so be sure not to mistake that feeling as withdrawal and choose whatever thirst-quenching option you fancy. Keeping yourself well hydrated is important for your physical and mental well-being. Thirst is your body telling you that it's not sufficiently hydrated and drinking water frequently and eating high water content foods such as fruit will make you feel great. Water is by far the best thirst-quencher and is freely available and if you want a hot drink then there are plenty of healthy, harmless ones to choose from. Naturally caffeine-free herb and fruit teas are fine. Rooibos (Redbush) tea, for example, naturally contains no caffeine.

Decaffeinated teas and coffees are those from which the caffeine has been artificially removed. The process of decaffeination itself has been found to create health problems and choosing these products also risks producing the feeling in your mind that you are substituting which can lead to a feeling of deprivation. So it's better to avoid them. Get it clear in your mind, you weren't drinking coffee, tea or energy drinks for the taste anyway. You were drinking them for the caffeine.

An amazing thing happens to your taste buds when you stop bombarding them with caffeine. They return to normal very quickly and you'll be able to enjoy the natural, more delicate and refined flavours in the drinks you do choose.

14. Enjoy breaking false associations. Whether it's during a break from sport or exercise, a break from work or from shopping, meeting a friend for a chat, or after a meal in a restaurant. These, and many others, are moments we've been brainwashed into automatically taking a caffeine product. It's great to purge the drug from your body and it's even more enjoyable breaking these associations. Feel happy to be free, knowing that you're in control. Enjoy these moments and think, "FANTASTIC! I'M FREE!"

15. Never envy caffeine addicts, pity them. Remember, they remain victims of the caffeine trap. They're wasting their money and time, harming their health and peace of mind, and diminishing their energy and vitality because of an addiction that provides them with no benefit whatsoever.

Watch people consuming caffeine while they're feeding their addiction. Does it look like they are enjoying some amazing treat?

If it appears to be relaxing them, see it for what it really is. A direct reaction to the level of anxiety and deprivation they were experiencing before that drink.

More often than not you will simply see a face of someone who isn't that interested in his or her drink and doesn't even seem to like the taste: a slave to the drug. The fact that they might remain oblivious to their predicament, and might remain so for the rest of their lives, is their loss. Would you envy someone who had a terrible illness but wasn't aware of it? Of course not. Get it clear in your mind, whenever you see anyone using caffeine, on any occasion, they're not doing it because they choose to, or want to, or because it gives them pleasure, or any kind of benefit, but because they've fallen for an ingenious, subtle confidence trick. Remember that you are not being deprived – they are. They're being deprived of their health, their money, their energy, their courage, their freedom. Consuming caffeine is nothing more or less than addiction to caffeine. You wouldn't envy a heroin addict.

You're free from the whole filthy nightmare.

ENJOY YOUR LIFE FREE FROM CAFFEINE!

THE INSTRUCTIONS THAT MAKE IT EASY TO QUIT

1. Cultivate the attitude "Isn't it great! My life is no longer affected by caffeine – I'm free!"

2. Never, ever doubt your decision: you know it's the right one and there's absolutely nothing to give up.

3. Do not – I repeat, do not – try to avoid thinking about caffeine.

4. Be aware that the little monster exists, but don't worry about him.

5. Don't worry if you occasionally forget that you've quit caffeine.

6. Check for caffeine in the ingredients of soft drinks, foods, snacks, and medications.

7. Don't wait to be a non-caffeine addict.

8. Accept that like everyone else on the planet you'll have good days and bad days.

9. Realize that you are in control of the craving and not the other way around.

10. Don't mourn the death of an enemy.

11. Don't change your life in any other way just because you quit caffeine.

12. Don't try to convert your friends unless they seek your help.

13. Don't use substitutes. Be wary of any thought process that implies any sense of deprivation. When you make choices think, "Great – I'll have…." rather than thinking you're missing out on something.

14. Always think: "FANTASTIC! I'M FREE!"

15. Never envy caffeine addicts.

TELL ALLEN CARR'S EASYWAY ORGANISATION THAT YOU'VE ESCAPED

Leave a comment on www.allencarr.com, like our Facebook page www.facebook.com/AllenCarr or write to the Worldwide Head Office address shown below.

ALLEN CARR'S EASYWAY CENTRES

The following list indicates the countries where Allen Carr's Easyway To Stop Smoking Centres are currently operational. Check www.allencarr.com for latest additions to this list. The success rate at the centres, based on the three-month money-back guarantee, is over 90 per cent.

Selected centres also offer sessions that deal with alcohol, other drugs, and weight issues. Please check with your nearest centre for details.

Allen Carr's Easyway guarantees that you will find it easy to stop at the centres or your money back.

ALLEN CARR'S EASYWAY

Worldwide Head Office
Park House, 14 Pepys Road, Raynes Park,
London SW20 8NH ENGLAND
Tel: +44 (0)208 9447761
Email: mail@allencarr.com
Website: www.allencarr.com

Worldwide Press Office

Tel: +44 (0)7970 88 44 52
Email: media@allencarr.com

UK Centre Information and Central Booking Line

0800 389 2115 (UK only)

UNITED KINGDOM	GERMANY	POLAND
	GREECE	PORTUGAL
REPUBLIC OF IRELAND	GUATEMALA	ROMANIA
	HONG KONG	RUSSIA
AUSTRALIA	HUNGARY	SAUDI ARABIA
AUSTRIA	IRAN	SERBIA
BAHRAIN	ISRAEL	SINGAPORE
BELGIUM	ITALY	SLOVENIA
BRAZIL	JAPAN	SOUTH AFRICA
BULGARIA	LEBANON	SOUTH KOREA
CANADA	MAURITIUS	SWEDEN
CHILE	MEXICO	SWITZERLAND
DENMARK	NETHERLANDS	TURKEY
ESTONIA	NEW ZEALAND	UAE
FINLAND	PERU	USA
FRANCE		

Visit www.allencarr.com to access your nearest centre's contact details.

OTHER ALLEN CARR PUBLICATIONS

Allen Carr's revolutionary Easyway method is available in a wide variety of formats, including digitally as audiobooks and ebooks, and has been successfully applied to a broad range of subjects. For more information about Easyway publications, please visit
shop.allencarr.com

Stop Smoking Now/Allen Carr's Quit Smoking Without Willpower

Stop Smoking with Allen Carr (with 70-minute audio CD)

Your Personal Stop Smoking Plan

Allen Carr's Quit Smoking Boot Camp

Finally Free!

The Easy Way for Women to Stop Smoking/Allen Carr's Easy Way for Women to Quit Smoking

The Illustrated Easy Way to Stop Smoking

The Illustrated Easy Way for Women to Stop Smoking

How to Be a Happy Non-Smoker

Smoking Sucks (Parent Guide with 16 page pull-out comic)

No More Ashtrays

The Little Book of Quitting Smoking

The Easy Way to Stop Smoking

The Easy Way to Control Alcohol

Your Personal Stop Drinking Plan

Stop Drinking Now / Allen Carr's Quit Drinking Without Willpower

The Illustrated Easy Way to Stop Drinking

The Easy Way for Women to Stop Drinking / Allen Carr's Easy Way for Women to Quit Drinking

No More Hangovers

Lose Weight Now

No More Diets

The Easy Way for Women to Lose Weight / Allen Carr's Easy Way for Women to Lose Weight

The Easy Way to Mindfulness

Good Sugar Bad Sugar

The Easy Way to Quit Sugar

The Easy Way to Stop Gambling

No More Debt

No More Worrying

The Easy Way to Enjoy Flying

Packing It In The Easy Way (the autobiography)

DISCOUNT VOUCHER FOR
ALLEN CARR'S EASYWAY CENTRES

Recover the price of this book when you
attend an Allen Carr's Easyway Centre
anywhere in the world.

Allen Carr has a global network of centres
where he guarantees you will find it easy to
stop smoking or your money back.

The success rate based on this money-back
guarantee is over 90 per cent.

When you book your appointment mention
this voucher and you will receive a discount
to the value of this book. Contact your
nearest centre for more information on
how the sessions work and to book your
appointment. Not valid in conjunction with
any other offer.